YOUR KNOWLEDGE HAS VALUE

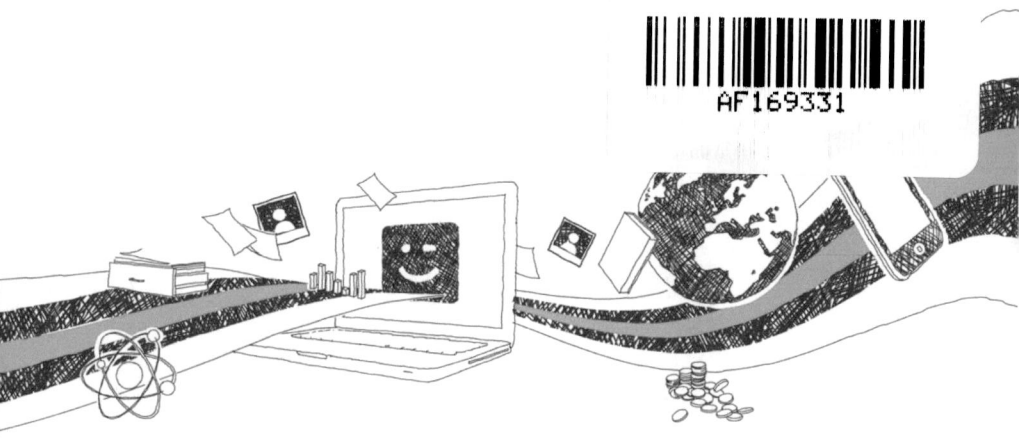

- We will publish your bachelor's and master's thesis, essays and papers

- Your own eBook and book - sold worldwide in all relevant shops

- Earn money with each sale

Upload your text at www.GRIN.com and publish for free

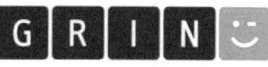

Bibliographic information published by the German National Library:

The German National Library lists this publication in the National Bibliography; detailed bibliographic data are available on the Internet at http://dnb.dnb.de .

This book is copyright material and must not be copied, reproduced, transferred, distributed, leased, licensed or publicly performed or used in any way except as specifically permitted in writing by the publishers, as allowed under the terms and conditions under which it was purchased or as strictly permitted by applicable copyright law. Any unauthorized distribution or use of this text may be a direct infringement of the author s and publisher s rights and those responsible may be liable in law accordingly.

Imprint:

Copyright © 2016 GRIN Verlag
Print and binding: Books on Demand GmbH, Norderstedt Germany
ISBN: 9783668826953

This book at GRIN:

https://www.grin.com/document/446734

Abubakar Sadiq Idris

Critical Analysis of the Socioeconomic Determinants of Malnutrition in Sub-Saharan Africa

GRIN Verlag

GRIN - Your knowledge has value

Since its foundation in 1998, GRIN has specialized in publishing academic texts by students, college teachers and other academics as e-book and printed book. The website www.grin.com is an ideal platform for presenting term papers, final papers, scientific essays, dissertations and specialist books.

Visit us on the internet:

http://www.grin.com/

http://www.facebook.com/grincom

http://www.twitter.com/grin_com

Faculty of Health and Life Sciences, Northumbria University

ABUBAKAR SADIQ IDRIS

Master of Public Health

Public Health Fundamentals: Concepts, Theories, and Frameworks

Year 1/2016

To be submitted on 13TH April, 2016

Content
Introduction 3
Poverty 4
Education 5
Government Policy and Political Will 7
Conclusion 9
References 10

CRITICAL ANALYSIS OF THE SOCIO-ECONOMIC DETERMINANTS OF MALNUTRITION IN SUB-SAHARAN AFRICA

Introduction

Malnutrition is a condition whereby normal bodily functions such as growth, physical activity, pregnancy, lactation, and immunity from diseases cannot be performed due to lack of appropriate nutrition (World Food Program (WFP), 2016). There are two forms; under nutrition and over nutrition (Robert et al, 2008) with under nutrition accounting for more than 33% of global infant mortality (Horton, 2014), in fact it is as high as 50% in some developing countries standing at over 50% and 40% in Nigeria and Ghana respectively (United Nations Children's Education Fund (UNICEF), 2016; Aheto et al., 2015). 795 million people all over the world are chronically malnourished with 780 million living in developing countries. The highest level globally is seen in sub-Saharan Africa with one in every four people being undernourished while only less than 5% of the population are affected in developed countries (FAO et al, 2015). Over nutrition on the other hand occurs when the diet consumed by an individual exceeds his nutrient requirement or the amount of calories needed to remain healthy (National Health Scheme (NHS), 2016), this has also been identified as a major public health problem seen majorly in developed countries (**Zukiewicz, 2014).**

Women and children are more commonly affected by malnutrition (Black et al, 2013). In fact one third of the annual global death of children is as a result of malnutrition, amounting to 2.6 million children (Robert et al, 2008). Despite the fact that the prevalence of malnutrition in sub-Saharan Africa have declined from 33.2% in 1990/92 to 23.2% in 2014/16, malnutrition still remains a challenge as the number of undernourished people in this region have actually increased due to high population growth rate (**World hunger and poverty facts and statistics (WHPS, 2015**). Despite the Significant progress made globally in improving food security and nutrition **(FAO, 2013),** same cannot be said for Sub-Saharan Africa **(Mabhaudhi, 2016)** as such it of paramount importance to identify the determinants that lead to malnutrition in this region in order to apply appropriate strategies to overcome them **(Raphael O. et al 2011).** UNICEF identified political, environmental, economic, social and cultural factors as the prime causes of under nutrition, noting that they are intricately connected to each other **(Robert et al, 2008).** It is however necessary to note that these determinants are quiet numerous and diverse, as such this essay will only focus on Poverty, lack of education, government policy and political will, at the same time attempt to show their interrelationship with each other and identify possible strategies to overcome them.

Poverty

There have been significant progress globally in reducing the level of extreme poverty since achieving the Millenium Development Goals (MDGS) target of reducing by half the global poverty rate in 2010. However, it has been estimated that 900 million people live below $1.9 a day in 2012 declining to 700 million people in 2015 which is still unacceptably high especially in sub-Saharan Africa which carried the largest global poverty burden (42.7%) in 2012 **(World Bank, 2016; WHPS, 2015).** Poverty is an important factor contributing to the lack of access to nutritious food, education, good health care and healthy living environment in sub-Saharan Africa, thus it sets a continuous trend of negative events **(Luchuo, 2013).** The number of people in extreme poverty in sub-Saharan Africa have been on the rise and this has been identified partly to be responsible for the degree of malnutrition **(WHPS, 2015).**

There is a strong correlation between the degree of malnutrition and household income, whereby households with low income have higher incidence of children with malnutrition as opposed to those with high income **(Luchuo, 2013; Raphael et al., 2011).** Most farmers in rural communities practice subsistence agriculture and do not have the capacity to access good agricultural machineries, fertilizers, storage fertilities and means of transportation due to poverty.

It has also been observed that children that suffer from malnutrition have poor cognitive and intellectual development in early childhood development resulting in poor classroom performance and subsequently grow to be less productive members of the society with resultant perpetuation of the poverty cycle in the community. This shows us one of the links between poverty and malnutrition, as such it has been hypothesized that breaking the cycle of malnutrition in early childhood will go a long way stopping inter-generational poverty in poor rural communities **(Mabhaudhi, 2016; Burchi, 2011).**

Most diet in sub-Saharan Africa is mainly cereal based with minor amount of proteins, vegetables and fruits. These foods are either too expensive to purchase, not available within their immediate environment or are just not considered as important as other pressing household needs **(Chastre, 2007)**.

Agriculture is the main source (70%) of food consumed by people in sub-Saharan Africa in addition to acting as a key source of livelihood and income. In fact, evidence suggests that improving income from agricultural production is more effective in reducing poverty and hunger when compared to other sectors, this is because poverty is seen more commonly in rural agricultural communities that rely more on agriculture for their survival **(Sassi, 2015; FAO, 2012; Livingston, 2011)**. This will in turn enhance food security and reduce malnutrition **(World Bank, 2008)**. This is further strenghthened by the fact that the level of undernutrition is negatively correlated to per capita income as such, economic empowerment is an effective way of improving the nutritional contents of diets and reducing the prevalence of malnutrition **(FAO, 2012)**.

Most communities in sub-Saharan Africa do not have access to basic amenities such as good sanitation facilities and hygienic water supply as such are predisposed to diseases such as cholera, diarrhea and intestinal worms which can ultimately lead to malnutrition or even death. **(Sassi, 2012, 2014)**. The world health organization identified diarrhea as the second leading cause of death in children under five years of age, killing about 760,000 children every year with over 1.7 billion cases annually. It has also been identified as the leading cause of malnutrition in children under five years of age. A significant proportion of diarrheal cases can be prevented with the provision of hygienic and safe drinking water, adequate sanitation and hygiene. However, these are not available to most communities in developing countries especially in sub-Saharan Africa **(WHO, 2013)**.

Education
One in every four children in sub-Saharan Africa is not in school, amounting to about 32 million children of primary school age, which represents 45% of the total out of school population globally and 54% of these children are girls. It has also been found that only one third of the youths attend secondary school and 38% of adults in sub-Saharan Africa cannot read or write with 60% of them being women **(UNESCO 2010)**. It has been estimated that in 2015, about 481 million women 15 years and over, do not have access to basic literacy skills, forming 64% of the

total number of people who are illiterate globally, a percentage that has remained unchanged since 2000, this shows us the extent of gender based inequalities in education especially in developing countries **(Galguera, 2015; UNESCO 2010).** Lack of education is a key factor with profound impact on nutrition, sanitation, personal hygiene and disease prevention techniques, all of which define the nutritional and health status and wellbeing of the community.

The inequity existing in most communities of sub-Saharan Africa in terms of educating the girl child and women is quite common and have profound influence on the level of nutrition of mothers and their children. In fact, evidence has shown that malnutrition is seen more often in children of less educated mothers. **(Ombati et al., 2012).** The Food and Agricultural Organization have also identified low birth weight, infant mortality, fatal diseases and weak classroom performance in children of malnourished pregnant or breastfeeding mothers **(Luchuo, 2013).**

Raphael et al. (2011) examined the prevalence and determinants of malnutrition among under five children in 40 farming communities in kwara state of Nigeria using descriptive and regression techniques to analyze anthropometrics data collected from children selected randomly. The result showed that 14.2% of the children were wasted, 22.0% were underweight and 23.6% were stunted. It also identified the major determinants of malnutrition in these children to include; gender and age of child, mother's education, calory intake of household, access to hygienic water supply as well as presence of toilets. A similar study carried out by **Aheto et al. (2015)** among under-five children in Ghana identified the risk factors for malnutrition to include; mothers education, economic status of the household, toilet facilities, multiple births, diarrheal disease and insurance coverage. These studies have shown the importance of mother's education to child's nutritional status, therefore in order to reduce the prevalence of malnutrition in these communities, there is need for programs that target girl child and women education in addition to provision of clean water supply, healthy sanitary and environmental conditions **(Ahetu et al. 2015; Raphael et al., 2011).**

However, **Deshmukh et al. (2012)** have also highlighted the importance of father's education in addition to that of the mother to child's nutrition, basing his argument on the fact that the father's educational level is a good indicator of his economic status and income which is directly to the family's ability to access adequate and nutritious food .

Malnutrition is seen in over 40% of school children in Nigeria and is responsible for 49% of absenteeism among primary school children. Based on this, the Nigerian government in 2005 in collaboration with New Partnership for African Development (NEPAD), World Food Program (WFP), and the United Nations International Children's Fund (UNICEF) developed the Home Grown School Feeding Health Program (HGSFHP). This program was aimed at reducing hunger among Nigerian children, improve their nutritional health status, increase school enrolment, retention and completion especially of children from rural communities. In addition, locally sourced food will be utilized, thus boosting the income of local farmers. However, Nigeria is yet to derive maximum benefits from this program as it is yet to be fully implemented as a national policy **(Yunusa, 2012)**.

In 2014 alone, the World Food Program provided school meals to 18.2 million children in 65 countries and supported nine other countries in their own school meals programmes **(WFP, 2014)**. This program is not only implemented in developing countries, even developed countries such as the United States of America, United Kingdom and Greece just to mention a few have introduced free breakfast schemes in both primary and secondary schools with resultant improvement in children's cognitive development and nutrition **(Harvey 2015; United States Department of Agriculture, 2015; Dimbley 2013)**.

Government Policy and Political Will

Most countries in sub-Saharan Africa have embraced democratic principles of governance. However, the challenges of poverty, corruption, debt, political instability, weak institutions, ethnic divisions and environmental disasters have stagnated development efforts **(NDI, 2016)**. Most sub-Saharan African countries have formulated policies aimed at improving agricultural production and reducing malnutrition, however a lot of flaws in these policies have led to their failure. A research by **Iwuchukwu and Igbokwe (2012)** in Nigeria noted some of the short comings to include; lack of strategy, targets and goals aimed at achieving results, lack of interaction with the required stakeholders in planning and implementation of policies, lack of continuity in government policies, conflict between different government programs, inconsistencies between regional and national policies, lack of monitoring and evaluation of such programs as well as corruption.

Possible ways of overcoming these policy deficiencies include; involvement of all stakeholders such as agricultural and economic experts down to the local farmers in the community in the process of planning, evaluation, implementation and monitoring of agricultural policies and programs. There should also be consistency in policies as well as providing the enabling environment for intra-regional trade and private sector participation in agricultural development. **(Iwuchukwu and Igbokwe (2012).**

Corruption is one of the major hindrances to the social, economic as well as health care development of Nigeria. Recent anti-corruption drive initiated by President Muhammadu Buhari upon assuming office in 2015 have exposed high profile individuals in corruption scandals involved in the theft or misappropriation of large sums of public money meant for developmental purposes. It has been estimated that if not appropriately controlled, corruption could cost Nigeria up to 37% of its Gross Domestic Product (GDP) by 2030 **(Price Water House Cooper (PWC), 2016).** Evidence have also shown the negative effect of corruption on food security and nutrition, as such there is need for government policy improvement in such a way that it will be more transparent, encourage accountability and discourage corruption. It should also enhance primary health care, improve food security, hygienic water supply, nutrition and education in order to control malnutrition and ensure growth and development in Nigeria and other sub-Saharan African Countries**(Uchendu and Olatunbosun, 2015).**

Many governments in sub-Saharan Africa have simply failed to assess the extent of malnutrition and its impact thus failing to consider the fight against it as important **(Luchuo, 2013).** The high level of malnutrition and food insecurity is also attributable to government's inability to provide appropriate infrastructure complicated by conflicts, infectious diseases and lack of access to health services **(Jessica, 2012).** Based on the fact that 95% of agricultural production is subsistence in nature and primarily depend on rainfall**(Singh, 2011)** improvement in irrigation infrastructure will result in improvement in agricultural production, food security and nutrition in poor rural communities. **(Mabhaudhi, 2016).**

"public policies should provide incentives for the adoption of sustainable agricultural intensification practices and techniques, sustainable land management, diversified agricultural systems and agro-forestry in order to produce more output from same area while reducing negative environmental inputs".

(FAO et al, 2015)

Reducing the number of undernourished people requires; making food available through domestic production, commercial imports and food assistance; improving access to food through economic empowerment, improved road networks as well as political stability; improving food utilization by provision of good sanitation and hygienic water supply. **(Sassi, 2015)**. However, **Mabhaudi (2016)** emphasized the need for a paradigm shift from focusing on these issues separately to approaching them as a single entity, thus encouraging interdisciplinary research between public health professionals, nutritionists, agricultural scientist and dieticians resulting in better recommendations that will empower policy makers to make a more informed decisions when formulating agricultural policies.

It has also been suggested that improvement in sub-regional co-operation and collaboration in terms of investments and policies as well as strong institutions, relevant and appropriate information is necessary for improvement in food security and economic growth(**Sassi, 2015**).

Conclusion
Malnutrition is a serious challenge posing tremendous negative impact in sub-Saharan Africa and the world in general. In view of this, the united nations (UN) proposed the Sustainable Development Goals (SDG2) which hopes to "End hunger, achieve food security and improved nutrition and ensure sustainable food production by 2030". Several socio-economic factors have been identified as the principal causes of malnutrition, some of these include poverty, lack of education, poor government policies, poor access to healthcare, poor access to hygienic water supply and environmental sanitation as well as access to toilet facilities, gender inequality and corruption. However, it is important to note that all of these factors are related to each other in one way or the other when it comes to causation of malnutrition. Thus, in order to mitigate the continued rise in the level of malnutrition in sub-Saharan Africa, a multifocal approach is needed. These factors should not be approached individually in the process of finding a viable

solution to the scourge of malnutrition; rather, they should be approached as a collective entity in the planning and implementation of government policies. This will in the long run ensure social justice and reduce societal inequalities with subsequent improvement in societal wellbeing, health and nutrition.

Governments must realize the huge socio-economic impact of malnutrition on the society and make good and appropriate policies with consideration of the prevailing conditions in the local communities when planning and implementing these policies.

References
Aheto, J. M. K., Keegan, T. J., Taylor, B. M., & Diggle, P. J. (2015). 'Childhood Malnutrition and Its Determinants among Under-Five Children in Ghana'. *Paediatric and perinatal epidemiology.* Volume *29, Issue* 6, pp.552-561. Doi: 10.1111/ppe.12222.

Black R. E, Cesar G V, Susan P. W, Zulfiqar A. B, Parul C., Mercedes D., Majid E., Sally G.,(2013), 'Maternal and child undernutrition and overweight in low-income and middle-income countries'. The Maternal and Child Nutrition Study Group 2013. *Lancet* Volume 382, No. 9890, pp.427–451.

Chastre, D., Duffield, A., Kindness, H., LeJeune S. and Taylor, A. (2007), 'The Minimum Cost of a Healthy Diet: Findings from Piloting a New Methodology in Four Study Locations', *Save the Children*: London UK.

Deshmukh, P. R., Sinha, N., & Dongre, A. R. (2013), 'Social determinants of stunting in rural area of Wardha, Central India'. *Medical Journal Armed Forces India*, Volume *69, Issue* 3, pp. 213-217.

Food and Agricultural Organization of the United Nations; Rome (2015). 'Meeting the 2015 international hunger targets: taking stock of uneven progress'. The state of food insecurity in the world. Available: http://www.fao.org/3/a4ef2d16-70a7-460a-a9ac-2a65a533269a/i4646e.pdf. Assessed 25 Feb 2016.

Food and Agricultural Organization of the United Nations; IFAD; WFP. 'The State of Food Insecurity in the World 2013: The Multiple Dimensions of Food Security', FAO: Rome, Italy, 2013.

Galguera, M. P. (2015); UNESCO (2015), 'Education for all 2000-2015: Achievements and Challenges. EFA Global Monitoring Report 2015, Paris, France.
Journal of Supranational Policies of Education (JOSPOE), Volume 3, pp.328-330. ISBN-978-92-3-10085-0.

Horton, S., Hoddinot, J.(2014). Food Security and Nutrition Perspective Paper: Benefits and Costs of the Food and Nutrition Targets for the Post-2015 Development Agenda; Copenhagen Consensus Center: Copenhagen, Denmark.

IFAD/FAD/FAO/WFP (2011), 'The state of food insecurity in the world', Rome, Italy: FAO Available:http://www.fao.org/docrep/014/i2330e/i2330e00.htm Assessed 26 Feb 2016.

Iwuchukwu J.C., Igbokwe E.M. (2012), 'Lessons from Agricultural Policies and Programmes in Nigeria', *Journal of Law, Policy and Globalization,* Vol 5, pp.12-18, ISSN 2224-3259.

Jessica Fanzo (2012). The nutritional challenge in sub-Saharan Africa', African Human Development Report of the United Nations Development Programme, Jan 2012. P. 26-35

Luchuo E. B., Paschal K, A Ngia Geraldine et al, (2013), 'Malnutrition in Sub-Saharan Africa: Burden, causes and prospects', *The Pan African Medical Journal*, Volume 15, Issue 120, Doi: 10.11604/pamj.2013.15.120.2535.

Mabhaudhi, T., Tendei, C., Albert, M. (2016), 'Water-Food-Nutrition Nexus: Linking Water to Improving Food, Nutrition and Health in Sub-Saharan Africa', *International Journal of Environmental Research and Public Health,* Vol. 13, No. 107; doi:10.3390/ijerf13010107.

National Health Scheme (2016), Obesity. Available: http://www.nhs.uk/Conditions/Obesity/Pages/Introduction.aspx, Accessed : 30th March, 2016.

National Democratic Institute (2016), 'Sub-Saharan Africa', Available: https://www.ndi.org/sub_saharan_africa, Accessed: 27 Feb 2016.

Ombati V., Mokua O. (2012),'Gender Inequity in Education in sub-Saharan Africa', *Academia*, UDC:37.043.1JEL:I2;I28, Available: https://www.academia.edu/6037312/Gender_Inequality_in_Education_in_sub_Saharan_AfricaA ccessed : 18 March, 2016.

Price Water House Cooper (2016), 'The Impact of Corruption on the Nigerian Economy'. Available: https://www.pwc.com/ng/en/assets/pdf/impact-of-corruption-on-nigerias-economy.pdf, Accessed: 1st April, 2016.

Raphael O.B, Segun B. F, Funke I. O, Foluke E. S. (2011), 'Prevalence and determinants of malnutrition among children of farming households in Kwara state, Nigeria'. *Journal of Agricultural Science,* Vol. 3, No.3, Doi:10.5539/jas.v3n3p173.

Robert E. B., L. H Allen, Z. A Bhutta, et al (2008), 'Maternal and Child Undernutrition: Global and Regional Exposures and Health Consequences', *The Lancet*, Jan 19 2008, 371(9608), 243-60, Available: DOI:10.1016/s0140-63736(07) 61690-0.

Sassi, M. (2015), 'A Spatial, Non-parametric Analysis of the Determinants of Food Insecurity in Sub-Saharan Africa', *African Development Review*, Vol. 27, No. 2, 2015, 92-105.

Uchendu F.,N., Olatunbosun, A., T. (2015),' Corrupt Practices Negatively Influence Food Security and Life Expectancy in Developing Countries', *Pan African Medical Journal,* Vol. 20, No. 110, pp.1-7, doi:10.11604/pamj.2015.20.110.5311.

United Nations Educational, Scientific and Cultural organization, "Education in Africa", Education for all global monitoring report (2010), Available: http://www.unesco.org/fileadmin/MULTIMEDIA/HQ/ED/GMR/pdf/gmr2010/aid-release-ssa-brief-en.pdf , Accessed: 28 Feb 2016.

United Nations, 'End hunger, achieve food security and improved nutrition and ensure sustainable agriculture', Millenium Development Goals, Available: http://www.un.org/sustainabledevelopment/hunger/, Accessed: 28th March, 2016.

United States Department of Agriculture Food and Nutrition Service, (2015), 'School Breakfast Program (SBP). Available: http://www.fns.usda.gov/sbp/school-breakfast-program-sbp, Accessed : 2nd April, 2016.

UNICEF (2015), Maternal and Child health: Nigeria, Available: http://www.unicef.org/nigeria/children_1926.html, Accessed: 30th March, 2016.

World Bank, "Agriculture for Development", World Development Report (2008), DOI: 10.1596/978-0-8213-7233-3.

World Bank (2016), Poverty and Equity; Sub-Saharan Africa. Available: http://povertydata.worldbank.org/poverty/region/SSA, Accessed : 30th March, 2016.

World Food Program (2014), 'School Meals', Available: http://documents.wfp.org/stellent/groups/public/documents/communications/wfp280714.pdf, Accessed: 31st March, 2016.

World Food Program (2016), 'What is malnutrition?' Available: https://www.wfp.org/hunger/malnutrition Accessed: 28 Feb 2016.

World Health Organization (2013), Diarrheal Disease Fact Sheet. Available: http://www.who.int/mediacentre/factsheets/fs330/en/ , Accessed : 31st March, 2016.

World hunger and poverty facts and statistics (2015), Available: http://worldhunger.org/articles/learn/world hunger facts 2002.htm Accessed: 30th March, 2016.

Yunusa, I., Gumel, A. M., Adegbusi, K., & Adegbusi, S. (2012). 'School feeding program in Nigeria: A vehicle for nourishment of pupils'. *The African Symposium: An Online Journal of African Educational Research Network.* Vol. 12, No. 2, pp. 104-110.

Zukiewicz-Sobczak, W., Wroblewska, P., Zwolinski, J., Chmielewska-Badora, J., Adamczuk, P., Krasowska, E., Zagorski, J., Oniszczuk, A., Piatek, J. and Silny, W., (2014). 'Obesity and poverty paradox in developed countries'. *Annals of Agricultural and Environmental Medicine*, Volume *21, Issue 3*.

YOUR KNOWLEDGE HAS VALUE

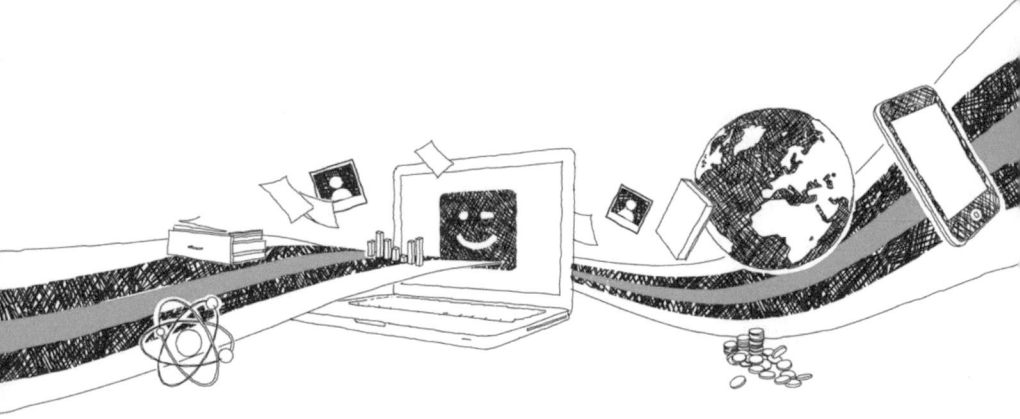

- We will publish your bachelor's and master's thesis, essays and papers

- Your own eBook and book - sold worldwide in all relevant shops

- Earn money with each sale

Upload your text at www.GRIN.com
and publish for free

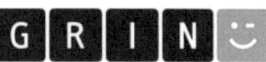